Delicious Air Fryer Recipes

Enjoy These Amazing Air Fryer Recipes for Daily Healthy Meals

Kira Hamm

TABLE OF CONTENT

Nugget and Veggie Taco Wraps

Preparation Time:5 minutes

Cooking Time: 15 minutes

Servings: 4

Ingredients:

- 1 tablespoon water
- 4pieces commercial vegan nuggets, chopped
- 1 small yellow onion, diced
- 1 small red bell pepper, chopped
- 2cobs grilled corn kernels
- 4large corn tortillas
- Mixed greens, for garnish

Directions:

1. Over a medium heat, sauté the nuggets in the water with the onion, corn kernels and bell pepper in a skillet, then remove from the heat.
2. Fill the tortillas with the nuggets and vegetables and fold them up. Transfer to the air fryer basket. Select the Air Fry function and cook at 400 degrees

Fahrenheit (204 degrees Celsius) for 15 minutes.

3. Once crispy, serve immediately, garnished with the mixed greens.

Nutrition: Calories 140 Fat 4g Fiber 3g Carbohydrates 5g Protein 7g

Cheesy Greens Sandwich

Preparation Time: 15 minutes

Cooking Time: 10 to 13 minutes

Servings: 4

Ingredients:

- 1½ cups chopped mixed greens
- 2garlic cloves, thinly sliced
- 2teaspoons olive oil
- 2slices low-sodium low-fat Swiss cheese
- 4slices low-sodium whole-wheat bread
- Cooking spray

Directions:

1. Select the Bake function and preheat Maxx to 400 degrees Fahrenheit (204 degrees Celsius).
2. In a baking pan, mix the greens, garlic, and olive oil. Bake for 4 to 5 minutes, stirring once, until the vegetables are tender. Drain, if necessary.
3. Make 2 sandwiches, dividing half of the greens and 1 slice of Swiss cheese between 2 slices of bread. Lightly spray the outsides of the sandwiches with cooking spray.

4. Bake the sandwiches in the air fryer oven for 6 to 8 minutes, turning with tongs halfway through, until the bread is toasted and the cheese melts.
5. Cut each sandwich in half and serve.

Nutrition: Calories 140 Fat 4g Fiber 3g Carbohydrates 5g Protein 7g

Cheesy Chicken Sandwich

Preparation Time:10 minutes

Cooking Time: 5 to 7 minutes

Servings: 1

Ingredients:

- 1/3 cup chicken, cooked and shredded
- 2Mozzarella slices
- 1 hamburger bun
- ¼ cup shredded cabbage
- 1 teaspoon mayonnaise
- 2teaspoons butter, melted
- 1 teaspoon olive oil
- ½ teaspoon balsamic vinegar
- ¼ teaspoon smoked paprika
- ¼ teaspoon black pepper
- ¼ teaspoon garlic powder
- Pinch of salt

Directions

1. Select the Bake function and preheat Maxx to 370 degrees Fahrenheit (188 degrees Celsius).
2. Brush some butter onto the outside of the hamburger bun.

3. In a bowl, coat the chicken with the garlic powder, salt, pepper, and paprika.
4. In a separate bowl, stir together the mayonnaise, olive oil, cabbage, and balsamic vinegar to make coleslaw.
5. Slice the bun in two. Start building the sandwich, starting with the chicken, followed by the Mozzarella, the coleslaw, and finally the top bun.
6. Transfer the sandwich to the air fryer oven and bake for 5 to 7 minutes.
7. Serve immediately.

Nutrition: Calories 311 Fat 11g Carbohydrate 22g Protein 31g

Lettuce Fajita Meatball Wraps

Preparation Time:10 minutes

Cooking Time: 10 minutes

Servings: 4

Ingredients:

- 1 pound (454 g) 85% lean ground beef
- ½ cup salsa, plus more for serving
- ¼ cup chopped onions
- ¼ cup diced green or red bell peppers
- 1 large egg, beaten
- 1 teaspoon fine sea salt
- ½ teaspoon chili powder
- ½ teaspoon ground cumin
- 1 clove garlic, minced
- Cooking spray
- For Serving:
- 8leaves Boston lettuce
- Pico de Gallo or salsa
- Lime slices

Directions

1. Spray the air fryer basket with cooking spray.

2. In a large bowl, mix together all the ingredients until well combined.
3. Shape the meat mixture into eight 1-inch balls. Place the meatballs in the air fryer basket, leaving a little space between them.
4. Select the Air Fry function and cook at 350 degrees Fahrenheit (177 degrees Celsius) for 10 minutes, or until cooked through and no longer pink inside and the internal temperature reaches 145 degrees Fahrenheit (63 degrees Celsius).
5. Serve each meatball on a lettuce leaf, topped with Pico de Gallo or salsa. Serve with lime slices.

Nutrition: Calories 576 Fat 49g Total Carbohydrates 8g Fiber 2g Protein 25g

Easy Homemade Hamburgers

Preparation Time:5 minutes

Cooking Time: 15 minutes

Servings: 2

Ingredients:

- 3/4-pound lean ground chuck
- Kosher salt and ground black pepper, to taste
- 3tablespoons onion, minced
- 1 teaspoon garlic, minced
- 1 teaspoon soy sauce
- 1/2 teaspoon smoked paprika
- 1/4 teaspoon ground cumin
- 1/2 teaspoon cayenne pepper
- 1/2 teaspoon mustard seeds
- 2burger buns

Directions:

1. Thoroughly combine the ground chuck, salt, black pepper, onion, garlic and soy sauce in a mixing dish.

2. Season with smoked paprika, ground cumin, cayenne pepper and mustard seeds. Mix to combine well.
3. Shape the mixture into 2 equal patties.
4. Spritz your patties with a nonstick cooking spray. Air fry your burgers at 380 degrees F for about 11 minutes or to your desired degree of doneness.
5. Place your burgers on burger buns and serve with favorite toppings. Devour!

Nutrition: Calories 433 Fat 17.4g Carbohydrates 40g Protein 39.2g Sugars 6.4g

Easy Beef Burritos

Preparation Time: 5 minutes

Cooking Time: 25 minutes

Servings: 3

Ingredients:

- 1 pound rump steak
- Sea salt and crushed red pepper, to taste
- 1/2 teaspoon shallot powder
- 1/2 teaspoon porcini powder
- 1/2 teaspoon celery seeds
- 1/2 teaspoon dried Mexican oregano
- 1 teaspoon piri Piri powder
- 1 teaspoon lard, melted
- 3(approx. 7-8" dia) whole-wheat tortillas

Directions:

1. Toss the rump steak with the spices and melted lard.
2. Cook in your Air Fryer at 390 degrees Fahrenheit for 20 minutes, turning it halfway through the cooking Time. Place on a cutting board to cool slightly.
3. Slice against the grain into thin strips.

4. Spoon the beef strips onto wheat tortillas; top with your favorite fixings, roll them up and serve. Enjoy!

Nutrition: Calories 368 Fat 13g Carbohydrates 20.2g Protein 35.1g Sugars 2.7g

Beef Parmigiana Sliders

Preparation Time:5 minutes

Cooking Time: 15 minutes

Servings: 2

Ingredients:

- 1/2-pound lean ground chuck
- 1 ounce bacon bits
- 2tablespoons tomato paste
- 3tablespoons shallots, chopped
- 1 garlic clove, minced
- 1/4 cup parmesan cheese, grated
- 1 teaspoon cayenne pepper
- Salt and black pepper, to taste
- 4pretzel rolls

Directions:

1. Thoroughly combine the ground chuck, bacon bits, tomato paste, shallots, garlic, parmesan cheese, cayenne pepper, salt, black pepper.
2. Shape the mixture into 4 equal patties.
3. Spritz your patties with a nonstick cooking spray. Air fry your burgers at 380 degrees

Fahrenheit for about 11 minutes or to your desired degree of doneness.

4. Place your burgers on pretzel rolls and serve with favorite toppings. Enjoy!

Nutrition: Calories 516 Fat 20.7g Carbohydrates 42g Protein 34.3g Sugars 5.1g

Chicago-Style Beef Sandwich

Preparation Time: 5 minutes

Cooking Time: 25 minutes

Servings: 2

Ingredients:

- 1/2-pound chuck, boneless
- 1 tablespoon olive oil
- 1 tablespoon soy sauce
- 1/4 teaspoon ground bay laurel
- 1/2 teaspoon shallot powder
- 1/4 teaspoon porcini powder
- 1/2 teaspoon garlic powder
- 1/2 teaspoon cayenne pepper
- Kosher salt and ground black pepper, to taste
- 1 cup pickled vegetables, chopped
- 2ciabatta rolls, sliced in half

Directions:

1. Toss the chuck roast with olive oil, soy sauce and spices until well coated.

2. Cook in the preheated Air Fryer at 400 degrees Fahrenheit for 20 minutes, turning over halfway through the cooking Time.
3. Shred the meat with two forks and adjust seasonings.
4. Top the bottom halves of the ciabatta rolls with a generous portion of the meat and pickled vegetables. Place the tops of the ciabatta rolls on the sandwiches. Serve immediately and enjoy!

Nutrition: Calories 385 Fat 17.4g Carbohydrates 28.1g Protein 29.8g Sugars 6.2g

Mediterranean Burgers with Onion Jam

Preparation Time: 5 minutes

Cooking Time: 25 minutes

Servings: 2

Ingredients:

- 1/2-pound ground chuck
- 2tablespoons scallions, chopped
- 1/2 teaspoon garlic, minced
- 1 teaspoon brown mustard
- 2Kosher salt and ground black pepper, to taste
- 2burger buns
- 2ounces Haloumi cheese
- 1 medium tomato, sliced
- Romaine lettuce leaves
- Onion jam:
- 2tablespoons butter, at room temperature
- red onions, sliced
- Sea salt and ground black pepper, to taste
- 2cup red wine
- tablespoons honey
- 2tablespoon fresh lemon juice

Directions:

1. Mix the ground chuck, scallions, garlic, mustard, salt and black pepper until well combined; shape the mixture into two equal patties.
2. Spritz a cooking basket with a nonstick cooking spray. Air fry your burgers at 370 degrees Fahrenheit for about 11 minutes or to your desired degree of doneness.
3. Meanwhile, make the onion jam. In a small saucepan, melt the butter; once hot, cook the onions for about 4 minutes. Turn the heat to simmer, add salt, black pepper and wine and cook until liquid evaporates.
4. Stir in the honey and continue to simmer until the onions are a jam-like consistency; afterwards, drizzle with freshly squeezed lemon juice.
5. Top the bottom halves of the burger buns with the warm beef patty. Top with haloumi cheese, tomato, lettuce and onion jam.
6. Set the bun tops in place and serve right now. Enjoy!

Nutrition: Calories 474 Fat 26.5g Carbohydrates

32.9g Protein 29g Sugars 26.1g

Italian Piadina Sandwich

Preparation Time:5 minutes

Cooking Time: 20 minutes

Servings: 2

Ingredients:

- 1/2-pound ribeye steak
- 1 teaspoon sesame oil
- Sea salt and red pepper, to taste
- 2medium-sized piadinas
- 2ounces Fontina cheese, grated
- 4tablespoons Giardiniera

Directions:

1. Brush the ribeye steak with sesame oil and season with salt and red pepper.
2. Cook at 400 degrees Fahrenheit for 6 minutes. Then, turn the steak halfway through the cooking Time and continue to cook for a further 6 minutes.
3. Slice the ribeye steak into bite-sized strips. Top the piadinas with steak strips and cheese.
4. Heat the sandwich in your Air Fryer at 380 degrees Fahrenheit for about 3 minutes

until the cheese melts. Top with Giardiniera and serve.

5. Bon appétit!

Nutrition: Calories 384 Fat 24.8g Carbohydrates 11.1g Protein 31.1g Sugars 4.9g

Taco Stuffed Avocados

Preparation Time:5 minutes

Cooking Time: 15 minutes

Servings: 2

Ingredients:

- 1/3-pound ground beef
- 2tablespoons shallots, minced
- 1/2 teaspoon garlic, minced
- 1 tomato, chopped
- 1/3 teaspoon Mexican oregano
- Salt and black pepper, to taste
- 1 chipotle pepper in adobo sauce, minced
- 1/4 cup cilantro
- avocados, cut into halves and pitted
- 1/2 cup Cotija cheese, grated

Directions:

1. Preheat a nonstick skillet over medium-high heat. Cook the ground beef and shallot for about 4 minutes.
2. Stir in the garlic and tomato and continue to sauté for a minute or so. Add in the Mexican oregano, salt, black pepper, chipotle pepper and cilantro.

3. Then, remove a bit of the pulp from each avocado half and fill them with the taco mixture.
4. Cook in the preheated Air Fryer at 400 degrees Fahrenheit for 5 minutes. Top with Cotija cheese and continue to cook for 4 minutes more or until cheese is bubbly. Enjoy!

Nutrition: Calories 521 Fat 42.1g Carbohydrates 23.1g Protein 20.2g Sugars 4.8g

Beef Taco Roll-Ups with Cotija Cheese

Preparation Time:5 minutes

Cooking Time: 25 minutes

Servings: 4

Ingredients:

- 1 tablespoon sesame oil
- 2tablespoons scallions, chopped
- 1 garlic clove, minced
- 1 bell pepper, chopped
- 1/2-pound ground beef
- 1/2 teaspoon Mexican oregano
- 1/2 teaspoon dried marjoram
- 1 teaspoon chili powder
- 1/2 cup refried beans
- Sea salt and ground black pepper, to taste
- 1/2 cup Cotija cheese, shredded
- 8roll wrappers

Directions:

1. Start by preheating your Air Fryer to 395 degrees Fahrenheit.
2. Heat the sesame oil in a nonstick skillet over medium-high heat. Cook the scallions,

garlic, and peppers until tender and fragrant.

3. Add the ground beef, oregano, marjoram, and chili powder. Continue cooking for 3 minutes longer or until it is browned.

4. Stir in the beans, salt, and pepper. Divide the meat/bean mixture between wrappers that are softened with a little bit of water. Top with cheese.

5. Roll the wrappers and spritz them with cooking oil on all sides.

6. Cook in the preheated Air Fryer for 11 to 12 minutes, flipping them halfway through the cooking Time. Enjoy!

Nutrition: Calories 417 Fat 15.9g Carbohydrates 41g Protein 26.2g Sugars 1.5g

Quick Sausage and Veggie Sandwiches

Preparation Time:5 minutes

Cooking Time: 35 minutes

Servings: 4

Ingredients:

- 4bell peppers
- 2tablespoons canola oil
- 4medium-sized tomatoes, halved
- 4spring onions
- 4beef sausages
- 4hot dog buns
- 1 tablespoon mustard

Directions:

1. Start by preheating your Air Fryer to 400 degrees Fahrenheit.
2. Add the bell peppers to the cooking basket. Drizzle 1 tablespoon of canola oil all over the bell peppers.
3. Cook for 5 minutes. Turn the temperature down to 350 degrees Fahrenheit. Add the tomatoes and spring onions to the cooking basket and cook an additional 10 minutes.

4. Reserve your vegetables.

5. Then, add the sausages to the cooking basket. Drizzle with the remaining tablespoon of canola oil.

6. Cook in the preheated Air Fryer at 380 degrees Fahrenheit for 15 minutes, flipping them halfway through the cooking Time.

7. Add the sausage to a hot dog bun; top with the air-fried vegetables and mustard; serve.

Nutrition: Calories 627 Fat 41.9g Carbohydrates 41.3g Protein 23.2g Sugars 9.3g

Cheesy Beef Burrito

Preparation Time:5 minutes

Cooking Time: 20 minutes

Servings: 4

Ingredients:

- 1 pound rump steak
- 1 teaspoon garlic powder
- 1/2 teaspoon onion powder
- 1/2 teaspoon cayenne pepper
- 1 teaspoon piri pudinas powder
- 1 teaspoon Mexican oregano
- Salt and ground black pepper, to taste
- 1 cup Mexican cheese blend
- 4large whole wheat tortillas
- 1 cup iceberg lettuce, shredded

Directions:

1. Toss the rump steak with the garlic powder, onion powder, cayenne pepper, piri pudinas powder, Mexican oregano, salt, and black pepper.
2. Cook in the preheated Air Fryer at 390 degrees Fahrenheit for 10 minutes. Slice

against the grain into thin strips. Add the cheese blend and cook for 2 minutes more.

3. Spoon the beef mixture onto the wheat tortillas; top with lettuce; roll up burrito-style and serve.

Nutrition: Calories 468 Fat 23.5g Carbohydrates 22.1g Protein 42.7g Sugars 2.3g

Burgers with Caramelized Onions

Preparation Time:5 minutes

Cooking Time: 30 minutes

Servings: 4

Ingredients:

- 1 pound ground beef
- Salt and ground black pepper, to taste
- 1 teaspoon garlic powder
- 1/2 teaspoon cumin powder
- 1 tablespoon butter
- 1 red onion, sliced
- 1 teaspoon brown sugar
- 1 tablespoon balsamic vinegar
- 1 tablespoon vegetable stock
- 4hamburger buns
- 8tomato slices
- 4teaspoons mustard

Directions:

1. Start by preheating your Air Fryer to 370 degrees Fahrenheit. Spritz the cooking basket with nonstick cooking oil.

2. Mix the ground beef with salt, pepper, garlic powder, and cumin powder. Shape the meat mixture into four patties and transfer them to the preheated Air Fryer.

3. Cook for 10 minutes; turn them over and cook on the other side for 8 to 10 minutes more.

4. While the burgers are frying, melt the butter in a pan over medium-high heat. Then, add the red onion and sauté for 4 minutes or until soft.

5. Add the brown sugar, vinegar, and stock and cook for 2 to 3 minutes more.

6. To assemble your burgers, add the beef patties to the hamburger buns. Top with the caramelized onion, tomato, and mustard. Serve immediately and enjoy!

Nutrition: Calories 475 Fat 21.1g Carbohydrates 33.3g Protein 36.2g Sugars 6.1g

Curried Shrimp and Zucchini Potstickers

Preparation Time: 35 minutes

Cooking Time: 5 minutes

Servings: 10

Ingredients:

- ½ pound peeled and deveined shrimp, finely chopped
- 1 medium zucchini, coarsely grated
- 1 tablespoon fish sauce
- 1 tablespoon green curry paste
- scallions, thinly sliced
- ¼ cup basil, chopped
- 30 round dumpling wrappers
- Cooking spray

Directions:

1. Combine the chopped shrimp, zucchini, fish sauce, curry paste, scallions, and basil in a large bowl. Stir to mix well.
2. Unfold the dumpling wrappers on a clean work surface, dab a little water around the edges of each wrapper, then scoop up 1

teaspoon of filling in the middle of each wrapper.

3. Make the potstickers: Fold the wrappers in half and press the edges to seal.
4. Spritz the perforated pan with cooking spray.
5. Transfer the potstickers to the pan and spritz with cooking spray.
6. Select Air Fry. Set temperature to 350 degrees Fahrenheit (180 degrees Celsius) and set Time to 5 minutes. Press Start to begin preheating.
7. Once preheated, place the pan into the oven. Flip the potstickers halfway through the cooking Time.
8. When cooking is complete, the potstickers should be crunchy and lightly browned.
9. Serve immediately.

Nutrition: Calories 347 Total Fat 7g Total Carbohydrates 44g Protein 22g

Cod Fish Tacos with Mango Salsa

Preparation Time:15 minutes

Cooking Time: 17 minutes

Servings: 6 tacos

Ingredients :

- 1 egg
- 5ounces Mexican beer
- ¾ cup all-purpose flour
- ¾ cup cornstarch
- ¼ teaspoon chili powder
- ½ teaspoon ground cumin
- ½ pound cod, cut into large pieces
- 6corn tortillas
- Cooking spray
- Salsa:
- 1 mango, peeled and diced
- ¼ red bell pepper, diced
- ½ small jalapeño, diced
- ¼ red onion, minced
- Juice of half a lime
- Pinch chopped fresh cilantro
- ¼ teaspoon salt

- ¼ teaspoon ground black pepper

Directions:

1. Spritz the perforated pan with cooking spray.

2. Whisk the egg with beer in a bowl. Combine the flour, cornstarch, chili powder, and cumin in a separate bowl.

3. Dredge the cod in the egg mixture first, then in the flour mixture to coat well. Shake the excess off.

4. Arrange the cod in the perforated pan and spritz with cooking spray.

5. Select Air Fry. Set temperature to 380 degrees Fahrenheit (193 degrees Celsius) and set Time to 17 minutes. Press Start to begin preheating.

6. Once preheated, place the pan into the oven. Flip the cod halfway through the cooking Time.

7. When cooked, the cod should be golden brown and crunchy.

8. Meanwhile, combine the Ingredients: for the salsa in a small bowl. Stir to mix well.

9. Unfold the tortillas on a clean work surface, then divide the fish on the tortillas and spread the salsa on top. Fold to serve.

Nutrition: Calories 126 Total Fat 12.1g Total Carbohydrates 2.8g Protein 2.1g

Bacon and Egg Wraps with Salsa

Preparation Time:15 minutes

Cooking Time: 10 minutes

Servings: 3

Ingredients:

- 3corn tortillas
- 3slices bacon, cut into strips
- 2scrambled eggs
- 3tablespoons salsa
- 1 cup grated Pepper Jack cheese
- 2tablespoons cream cheese, divided
- Cooking spray

Directions:

1. Spritz the perforated pan with cooking spray.
2. Unfold the tortillas on a clean work surface, divide the bacon and eggs in the middle of the tortillas, then spread with salsa and scatter with cheeses. Fold the tortillas over.
3. Arrange the tortillas in the pan.

4. Select Air Fry. Set temperature to 390 degrees Fahrenheit (199 degrees Celsius) and set Time to 10 minutes. Press Start to begin preheating.
5. Once the oven has preheated, place the pan into the oven. Flip the tortillas halfway through the cooking Time.
6. When cooking is complete, the cheeses will be melted and the tortillas will be lightly browned.
7. Serve immediately.

Nutrition: Calories 290 Total Fat 10.5g Total Carbohydrates 23.2g Protein 27.3g

Chicken Wraps with Ricotta Cheese

Preparation Time:30 minutes

Cooking Time: 5 minutes

Servings: 12

Ingredients:

1. 2large-sized chicken breasts, cooked and shredded
2. 2spring onions, chopped
3. 10ounces (284 g) Ricotta cheese
4. 1 tablespoon rice vinegar
5. 1 tablespoon molasses
6. 1 teaspoon grated fresh ginger
7. ¼ cup soy sauce
8. 1/3 teaspoon sea salt
9. ¼ teaspoon ground black pepper, or more to taste
10.   48 wonton wrappers
11.   Cooking spray

Directions:

1. Spritz the perforated pan with cooking spray.

2. Combine all the ingredients, except for the wrappers in a large bowl. Toss to mix well.

3. Unfold the wrappers on a clean work surface, then divide and spoon the mixture in the middle of the wrappers.

4. Dab a little water on the edges of the wrappers, then fold the edge close to you over the filling. Tuck the edge under the filling and roll up to seal.

5. Arrange the wraps in the pan.

6. Select Air Fry. Set temperature to 375 degrees Fahrenheit (190 degrees Celsius) and set Time to 5 minutes. Press Start to begin preheating.

7. Once preheated, place the pan into the oven. Flip the wraps halfway through the cooking Time.

8. When cooking is complete, the wraps should be lightly browned.

9. Serve immediately.

Nutrition: Calories 250 Total Fat 10.1g Total Carbohydrates 4.9g Protein 34.2g

Sweet Potato and Spinach Burritos

Preparation Time:15 minutes

Cooking Time: 30 minutes

Servings: 6 burritos

Ingredients:

- 2sweet potatoes, peeled and cut into a small dice
- 1 tablespoon vegetable oil
- Kosher salt and ground black pepper, to taste
- 6large flour tortillas
- 1 (16-ounce) can refried black beans, divided
- 1 ½ cups baby spinach, divided
- 6eggs, scrambled
- ¾ cup grated Cheddar cheese, divided
- ¼ cup salsa
- ¼ cup sour cream
- Cooking spray

Directions:

1. Put the sweet potatoes in a large bowl, then drizzle with vegetable oil and sprinkle with salt and black pepper. Toss to coat well.
2. Place the potatoes in the perforated pan.
3. Select Air Fry. Set temperature to 400 degrees Fahrenheit (205 degrees Celsius) and set Time to 10 minutes. Press Start to begin preheating.
4. Once preheated, place the pan into the oven. Flip the potatoes halfway through the cooking Time.
5. When done, the potatoes should be lightly browned. Remove the potatoes from the oven.
6. Unfold the tortillas on a clean work surface. Divide the black beans, spinach, air fried sweet potatoes, scrambled eggs, and cheese on top of the tortillas.
7. Fold the long side of the tortillas over the filling, then fold in the shorter side to wrap the filling to make the burritos.
8. Wrap the burritos in the aluminum foil and put in the pan.

9. Select Air Fry. Set temperature to 350 degrees Fahrenheit (180 degrees Celsius) and set Time to 20 minutes. Place the pan into the oven. Flip the burritos halfway through the cooking Time.

10. Remove the burritos from the oven and spread with sour cream and salsa. Serve immediately.

Nutrition: Calories 385 Total Fat 9g Total Carbohydrates 32g Protein 13g

Cabbage and Prawn Wraps

Preparation Time:20 minutes

Cooking Time: 18 minutes

Servings: 4

Ingredients:

- 2tablespoons olive oil
- 1 carrot, cut into strips
- 1-inch piece fresh ginger, grated
- 1 tablespoon minced garlic
- 2tablespoons soy sauce
- ¼ cup chicken broth
- 1 tablespoon sugar
- 1 cup shredded Napa cabbage
- 1 tablespoon sesame oil
- 8cooked prawns, minced
- 8egg roll wrappers
- 1 egg, beaten
- Cooking spray

Directions:

1. Spritz the perforated pan with cooking spray. Set aside.

2. Heat the olive oil in a nonstick skillet over medium heat until shimmering.

3. Add the carrot, ginger, and garlic and sauté for 2 minutes or until fragrant.

4. Pour in the soy sauce, broth, and sugar. Bring to a boil. Keep stirring.

5. Add the cabbage and simmer for 4 minutes or until the cabbage is tender.

6. Turn off the heat and mix in the sesame oil. Let sit for 15 minutes.

7. Use a strainer to remove the vegetables from the liquid, then combine with the minced prawns.

8. Unfold the egg roll wrappers on a clean work surface, then divide the prawn mixture in the center of wrappers.

9. Dab the edges of a wrapper with the beaten egg, then fold a corner over the filling and tuck the corner under the filling. Fold the left and right corner into the center. Roll the wrapper up and press to seal. Repeat with remaining wrappers.

10. Arrange the wrappers in the pan and spritz with cooking spray.

11. Select Air Fry. Set temperature to 370 degrees Fahrenheit (188 degrees Celsius) and set Time to 12 minutes. Press Start to begin preheating.

12. Once the oven has preheated, place the pan into the oven. Flip the wrappers halfway through the cooking Time.

13. When cooking is complete, the wrappers should be golden.

14. Serve immediately.

Nutrition: Calories 339 Total Fat 15.9g Total Carbohydrates 27.5g Protein 24.2g

Ricotta Spinach and Basil Pockets

Preparation Time:20 minutes

Cooking Time: 10 minutes

Servings: 8 pockets

Ingredients:

- 2large eggs, divided
- 1 tablespoon water
- 1 cup baby spinach, roughly chopped
- ¼ cup sun-dried tomatoes, finely chopped
- 1 cup ricotta cheese
- 1 cup basil, chopped
- ¼ teaspoon red pepper flakes
- ¼ teaspoon kosher salt
- 2refrigerated rolled pie crusts
- 2tablespoons sesame seeds

Directions:

- Spritz the perforated pan with cooking spray.
- Whisk an egg with water in a small bowl.
- Combine the spinach, tomatoes, the other egg, ricotta cheese, basil, red pepper

flakes, and salt in a large bowl. Whisk to mix well.

- Unfold the pie crusts on a clean work surface and slice each crust into 4 wedges. Scoop up 3 tablespoons of the spinach mixture on each crust and leave ½ inch space from edges.
- Fold the crust wedges in half to wrap the filling and press the edges with a fork to seal.
- Arrange the wraps in the pan and spritz with cooking spray. Sprinkle with sesame seeds.
- Select Air Fry. Set temperature to 380 degrees Fahrenheit (193 degrees Celsius) and set Time to 10 minutes. Press Start to begin preheating.
- Once the oven has preheated, place the pan into the oven. Flip the wraps halfway through the cooking Time.
- When cooked, the wraps will be crispy and golden.
- Serve immediately.

Nutrition: Calories 175 Total Fat 13.4g Total

Carbohydrates 2g Protein 11.9g

Avocado and Tomato Wraps

Preparation Time: 10 minutes

Cooking Time: 5 minutes

Servings: 5

Ingredients:

- 10egg roll wrappers
- 3avocados, peeled and pitted
- 1 tomato, diced
- Salt and ground black pepper, to taste
- Cooking spray

Directions:

1. Spritz the perforated pan with cooking spray.

2. Put the tomato and avocados in a food processor. Sprinkle with salt and ground black pepper. Pulse to mix and coarsely mash until smooth.

3. Unfold the wrappers on a clean work surface, then divide the mixture in the center of each wrapper. Roll the wrapper up and press to seal.

4. Transfer the rolls to the pan and spritz with cooking spray.

5. Select Air Fry. Set temperature to 350 degrees Fahrenheit (180 degrees Celsius) and set Time to 5 minutes. Press Start to begin preheating.

6. Once the oven has preheated, place the pan into the oven. Flip the rolls halfway through the cooking Time.

7. When cooked, the rolls should be golden brown.

8. Serve immediately.

Nutrition: Calories 419 Total Fat 14g Total Carbohydrates 39g Protein 33g

Hot Bacon Sandwiches

Preparation Time:10 minutes

Cooking Time: 7 minutes

Servings: 4

Ingredients:

- 1/3 cup BBQ sauce
- 8bacon slices, cooked and cut into thirds
- 1 red bell pepper, sliced
- 2tablespoon honey
- butter
- 1 and ¼ cup lettuce leaves, torn
- 3pita pockets, halved
- 8tomatoes, sliced
- 1 yellow bell pepper, sliced

Directions:

1. Mix honey and BBQ sauce in a bowl and whisk properly.
2. Brush bell peppers and bacon with some of this mixture
3. Set them in your air fryer, and cook for around 4 minutes at 350 degrees Fahrenheit

4. Shaking the fryer and cook them for about 2 minutes extra.
5. Stuff pita pockets with bacon mix, and also stuff with lettuce and tomatoes.
6. Expand the bottom of the BBQ sauce and serve them for lunch.

Nutrition: Calories 186 Fiber 9g Carbohydrates 14g Fat 6g Protein 4g

Chicken Sandwiches

Preparation Time:10 minutes

Cooking Time: 10 minutes

Servings: 4

Ingredients:

- 2chicken breasts, skinless, boneless and cubed
- 1 red bell pepper, sliced
- 1 red onion, chopped
- ½ teaspoon thyme, dried
- ½ cup Italian seasoning
- 2cups butter lettuce, torn
- 4pita pockets
- 1 tablespoon olive oil
- 1 cup cherry tomatoes, halved

Directions:

1. Mix chicken with bell pepper, onion, oil, and Italian seasoning in your air fryer, toss well, and cook for 10 minutes at 380 degrees Fahrenheit.
2. Transfer the mixture to a bowl, add butter, lettuce, thyme, cherry, tomatoes, and toss well.

3. Stuff pita pockets with the mixture and then serve them for lunch.

Nutrition: Calories 126 Fiber 8g Carbohydrates 14g Fat 4g Protein 4g

Easy Hot Dogs

Preparation Time:10 minutes

Cooking Time: 7 minutes

Servings: 2

Ingredients:

- 2hot dog buns
- Dijon mustard (1 tablespoon)
- 2hot dogs
- cheddar cheese, grated (2 tablespoons)

Directions:

1. Put hot dogs in the preheated air fryer and cook them for around 5 minutes at 390 degrees Fahrenheit.
2. Arrange hot dogs into the hot dog buns, expand cheese, and mustard.
3. Return everything to the air fryer and cook at 390 degrees Fahrenheit for 2 minutes extra.
4. Serve them for lunch.

Nutrition: Calories 211 Fiber 8g Carbohydrates 12g Fat 3g Protein 4g

Turkey Burgers

Preparation Time: 10 minutes

Cooking Time: 8 minutes

Servings: 4

Ingredients:

- 1 shallot, minced
- 1 pound turkey meat, ground
- Zest from 1 lime, grated
- 1 small jalapeno pepper, minced
- 2teaspoons lime juice
- A drizzle of olive oil
- black pepper and salt
- 1 teaspoon cumin, ground
- Guacamole for serving
- 1 teaspoon sweet paprika

Directions:

1. Mix turkey meat with pepper, cumin, paprika, jalapeno, lime juice, shallot, and zest in a bowl, stir well, shape burgers from this mix, drizzle the oil over them, introduce in the preheated air fryer and cook them for around 8 minutes on all side at 370 degrees Fahrenheit.

2. Distribute between plates and serve them with guacamole on top.

Nutrition: Calories 200 Fiber 0g Carbohydrates 0g Fat 12g Protein 12g

Prosciutto Sandwich

Preparation Time: 10 minutes

Cooking Time: 5 minutes

Servings: 1

Ingredients:

1. 2mozzarella slices
2. 1 teaspoon olive oil
3. 2bread slices
4. 2prosciutto slices
5. 2tomato slices
6. 2basil leaves
7. A pinch of black pepper and salt

Directions:

1. Arrange prosciutto and mozzarella on a bread piece.
2. Season with pepper and salt, put them in your air fryer, and cook for 5 minutes at 400 degrees Fahrenheit.
3. Drizzle oil above prosciutto, add basil and tomato cover with the other bread piece, chopped sandwich in half and serve them.
4. Enjoy!

Nutrition: Calories 172 Fiber 7g Carbohydrates 9g Fat

3g Protein 5g

Tasty Cheeseburgers

Preparation Time: 10 minutes

Cooking Time: 20 minutes

Servings: 2

Ingredients:

- teaspoons
- 4cheddar cheese slices
- 2teaspoons
- 12ounces lean beef, ground
- 2tablespoons yellow onion, chopped
- black pepper and salt
- 2burger buns, halved

Directions:

1. Mix beef with ketchup, salt mustard, onion, and pepper in a bowl; stir well and shape four patties out of the mixture.
2. Arrange cheese on two patties and the top with another two patties.
3. Put them in a preheated air fryer at 370 degrees Fahrenheit and stir-fry them for around 20 minutes.

4. Place the cheeseburger on two bread bun halves, and the top with another two halves, and serve for lunch.

Nutrition: Calories 261 Fiber 10g Carbohydrates 20g Fat 6g Protein 6g

Rolled Salmon Sandwich

Preparation Time: 5 minutes

Cooking Time: 5 minutes

Servings: 1

Ingredients:

- 1 piece of flatbread
- 1 salmon filet
- Pinch of salt
- 1 tablespoon green onion, chopped
- 1/4 teaspoon dried sumac
- 1/2 teaspoon thyme
- 1/2 teaspoon sesame seeds
- 1/4 English cucumber
- 1 tablespoon yogurt

Directions:

1. Start by peeling and chopping the cucumber. Cut the salmon at a 45-degree angle into 4 slices and lay them flat on the flatbread.
2. Sprinkle salmon with salt to taste. Sprinkle onions, thyme, sumac, and sesame seeds evenly over the salmon.

3. Broil the salmon for at least 3 minutes, but longer if you want a more well-done fish.

4. While you broil your salmon, mix the yogurt and cucumber. Remove your flatbread from the toaster oven, put it on a plate, and spoon the yogurt mix over the salmon.

5. Fold the flatbread sides in and roll it up for a gourmet lunch that you can take on the go.

Nutrition: Calories 347 Sodium 397mg Dietary Fiber 1.6g Total Fat 12.4g Total Carbohydrates 20.6g Protein 38.9g

Chicken Capers Sandwich

Preparation Time:3 minutes

Cooking Time: 3 minutes

Servings: 2

Ingredients:

- 2leftover chicken breasts or pre-cooked breaded chicken
- 1 large ripe tomato
- 2ounces' mozzarella cheese slices
- 3slices of whole-grain bread
- 1/4 cup olive oil
- 1/3 cup fresh basil leaves
- Salt and pepper to taste

Directions:

1. Start by slicing tomatoes into thin slices.
2. Layer tomatoes, then cheese over two slices of bread and place on a greased baking sheet.
3. Grill for about 3 minutes
4. Heat chicken while the cheese melts.
5. Remove from oven, sprinkle with basil, and add chicken.
6. Sprinkle with oil and add salt and pepper.

7. Top with other slices of bread and serve.

Nutrition: Calories 808 Sodium 847mg Dietary Fiber 5.2g Total Fat 43.6g Total Carbohydrates 30.7g Protein 78.4g

Easy Prosciutto Grilled Cheese

Preparation Time: 5 minutes

Cooking Time: 5 minutes

Servings: 1

Ingredients:

- 2slices muenster cheese
- 2slices white bread
- 2thinly-shaved pieces of prosciutto
- 1 tablespoon sweet and spicy pickles

Directions:

1. Set air fryer oven to the Toast setting.
2. Put one slice of cheese on each piece of bread.
3. Put prosciutto on one slice and pickles on the other.
4. Take it to a baking sheet and toast for 4 minutes or until the cheese is melted.
5. Combine the sides, cut, and serve.

Nutrition: Calories 460 Sodium 2180mg Dietary Fiber 0g Total Fat 25.2g Total Carbohydrates 11.9g Protein 44.2g

Persimmon Toast with Sour Cream and Cinnamon

Preparation Time:5 minutes

Cooking Time: 5 minutes

Servings: 1

Ingredients:

- 1 slice of wheat bread
- 1/2 persimmon
- Sour cream to taste
- Sugar to taste
- Cinnamon to taste

Directions:

1. Apply a thin layer of sour cream across the bread.
2. Slice the persimmon into 1/4-inch pieces and lay them across the bread.
3. Sprinkle cinnamon and sugar over persimmon.
4. Toast in the air fryer oven until bread and persimmon begin to brown.

Nutrition: Calories 89 Sodium 133mg Dietary Fiber 2.0g Total Fat 1.1g Total Carbohydrates 16.5g Protein 3.8g

Roasted Grape and Goat Cheese Crostinis

Preparation Time: 30 minutes

Cooking Time: 5 minutes

Servings: 10

Ingredients:

- 1-pound seedless red grapes
- 1 teaspoon chopped rosemary
- 2tablespoons olive oil
- 1 rustic French baguette
- 1 cup sliced shallots
- 2tablespoons unsalted butter
- 2ounces' goat cheese
- 1 tablespoon honey

Directions:

1. Start by preheating the air fryer oven to 400 degrees Fahrenheit.
2. Toss grapes, rosemary, and 1 tablespoon of olive oil in a large bowl.
3. Take it to a roasting pan and roast for 20 minutes.
4. Remove the pan from the oven and set aside to cool.

5. Slice the baguette into 1/2-inch-thick pieces.

6. Rub each slice with olive oil and place on a baking sheet.

7. Cook for 8 minutes, then remove from oven and set aside.

8. In a medium skillet, add butter and one tablespoon of olive oil.

9. Add shallots and sauté for about 10 minutes.

10. Mix goat cheese and honey in a medium bowl, then add the shallot pan and mix thoroughly.

11. Spread shallot mixture onto a baguette, top with grapes, and serve.

Nutrition: Calories 238 Sodium 139mg Dietary Fiber 0.6g Total Fat 16.3g Total Carbohydrates 16.4g Protein 8.4g

Veggies on Toast

Preparation Time:12 minutes

Cooking Time: 11 minutes

Servings: 4

Ingredients:

- 1 red bell pepper, cut into ½-inch strips
- 1 cup sliced button or cremini mushrooms
- 1 small yellow squash, sliced
- 2green onions, cut into ½-inch cuts
- Extra light olive oil
- 3to 6 pieces sliced French bread
- 2tablespoons softened butter
- ½ cup soft goat cheese

Directions:

1. Mix the red pepper, mushrooms, squash, and green onions in the air fryer and mist with oil.
2. Cook for 15 minutes until the vegetables are tender, shaking the basket once during cooking Time.
3. Take out the vegetables from the basket and set aside.

4. Put the bread with butter and place in the air fryer.
5. Heat up for 2 to 4 minutes or until golden brown.
6. Put the goat cheese on the toasted bread and top with the vegetables; serve warm.

Nutrition: Calories 162 Sodium 160mg Fiber 2g Total Fat 11g Saturated Fat 7g Carbohydrates 9g Protein 7g Cholesterol 30mg

Mushroom Pita Pizzas

Preparation Time: 10 minutes

Cooking Time: 5 minutes

Servings: 4

Ingredients:

- 4(3-inch) pitas
- 1 tablespoon olive oil
- ¾ cup pizza sauce
- 1 (4-ounce) jar sliced mushrooms, drained
- ½ teaspoon dried basil
- 2green onions, minced
- 1 cup grated mozzarella or provolone cheese
- 1 cup sliced grape tomatoes

Directions:

1. Put each piece of pita with oil and top with the pizza sauce.
2. Put the mushrooms and sprinkle with basil and green onions. Put with the grated cheese.
3. Bake for 5 to 10 minutes or until the cheese is melted and starts to brown. Put with the grape tomatoes.

Nutrition: Calories 231 Sodium 500mg Fiber 2g Total Fat 9g Saturated Fat 4g Carbohydrates 25g Protein 13g Cholesterol 15mg

French Toast Sticks with Sugar and Berries

Preparation Time:10 Minutes

Cooking Time: 10 Minutes

Servings: 4

Ingredients:

- 4(2-inch thick) bread slices
- 2large eggs
- ¼ cup whole milk
- ¼ cup brown sugar
- 1 tbsp maple syrup
- 1 tsp cinnamon powder
- A pinch nutmeg powders
- pinches icing sugar for topping
- 2Fresh blueberries and raspberries for topping

Directions:

1. Insert the drip pan at the bottom rack of the device and preheat the air fryer at Air Fryer mode at 350 degrees Fahrenheit for 3 to 4 minutes.

2. Cut each bread slice into 4 long strips and set aside.

3. Open the eggs into a bowl then whisk in the milk, maple syrup, cinnamon powder, and nutmeg powder.
4. Place the cooking tray to your side. Working in batches, dip 7 to 8 bread strips into the egg mixture and arrange widthwise on the tray.
5. Open the oven and fit in the cooking tray on the middle rack. Set the Timer for 10 minutes, then cook until the Timer reads to the end.
6. Open the oven, remove the tray and check the toasts, which should not be wet but crispy and sweet.
7. Transfer to serving plates and make the remaining toasts.
8. To serve, sprinkle with the icing sugar and enjoy warm with the berries.

Nutrition: Calories 132 Total Fat 4g Total Carbohydrates 17.12g Fiber 1.7g Protein 6.77g Sugar 3.82g Sodium 190mg

Coconut Sandwich with Tomato and Avocado

Preparation Time: 5 Minutes

Cooking Time: 15 Minutes

Servings: 4

Ingredients:

- ½ cup almond flour
- ¼ teaspoon salt
- ¼ teaspoon baking soda
- 2 eggs
- 2 tablespoons coconut oil
- 2 tablespoons coconut milk
- 1 ripe avocado
- 1 large red tomato

Directions:

1. Combine the almond flour with salt and baking soda then mix well.
2. Make a hole in the center of the flour mixture then add eggs, coconut oil, and coconut milk to it. Stir until incorporated.
3. Line a baking pan that fits the Kalorik Maxx Air Fryer Oven then grease it with cooking spray.

4. Transfer the batter to the baking pan and spread it evenly.

5. Next, install the crisper plate into the basket of your Kalorik Maxx Air Fryer Oven then preheat the for 3 minutes.

6. Select the "Bake" menu then set the temperature to 325 degrees Fahrenheit and adjust the Time to 10 minutes.

7. Insert the baking pan to the Kalorik Maxx's basket then press the "Start/Stop" button to begin. Bake the bread.

8. Once the Kalorik Maxx beeps and the bread is done, remove it from the Kalorik Maxx and take the bread out of the pan.

9. Cut the bread into thick slices then top each slice of bread with avocado and tomato slices.

10.   Serve and enjoy.

Nutrition: 242 Calories, 22.6g Fats, 2.9g Net Carbs, 5g Protein

Avocado Taco Fry

Preparation Time: 5 Minutes

Cooking Time: 20 Minutes

Servings: 12

Ingredients:

- 1 peeled avocado, sliced
- 1 beaten egg
- 1/2 cup panko bread crumbs
- Salt
- Tortillas and toppings

Directions:

1. Using a bowl, add in the egg.
2. Using a separate bowl, set in the breadcrumbs.
3. Dip the avocado into the bowl with the beaten egg and coat with the breadcrumbs. Sprinkle the coated wedges with a bit of salt.
4. Arrange them in the cooking basket in a single layer.
5. Set the Air Fryer to 392 degrees Fahrenheit and cook for 15 minutes. Shake the basket halfway through the cooking process.

6. Put them on tortillas with your preferred toppings.

Nutrition: Calories 140 Fat 8.8g Carbohydrates 12g Protein 6g

Scallion Sandwich

Preparation Time: 10 Minutes

Cooking Time: 15 Minutes

Servings: 1

Ingredients:

- 2slices of wheat bread
- 2tsp. low-fat butter
- 2sliced scallions
- 1 tbsp. grated parmesan cheese
- 3/4 cup low-fat, grated cheddar cheese

Directions:

1. Adjust the Air fryer to 356 degrees Fahrenheit.
2. Apply butter to a slice of bread. Then place it inside the cooking basket with the butter side facing down.
3. Place cheese and scallions on top. Spread the rest of the butter on the other slice of bread. Then put it on top of the sandwich and sprinkle with parmesan cheese.
4. Allow cooling for 10 minutes. Serve.

Nutrition: Calories 154 Fat 2.5g Carbohydrates 9g Protein 8.6g

Breakfast Cheese Bread Cups

Preparation Time:6 Minutes

Cooking Time: 15 Minutes

Servings: 2

Ingredients:

1. 2eggs
2. 2tbsps. grated cheddar cheese
3. Salt and pepper
4. 1 ham slice cut into two pieces
5. 4bread slices flatted with a rolling pin
6. Directions:
7. Spray both sides of the ramekins with cooking spray.
8. Place two slices of bread into each ramekin.
9. Add the ham slice pieces into each ramekin.
10. Crack an egg in each ramekin, then sprinkle with cheese.
11. Season with salt and pepper.
12. Place the ramekins into the air fryer at 300 degrees Fahrenheit for 15 minutes.

13. Serve warm.

Nutrition: Calories 162 Total Fat 8g Carbohydrates 10g Protein 11g

Cheese and Egg Breakfast Sandwich

Preparation Time:3 Minutes

Cooking Time: 6 Minutes

Servings: 1

Ingredients:

- 1 egg
- 2slices of cheddar or Swiss cheese
- A bit of butter
- 1 roll either English muffin or Kaiser bun halved

Directions:

1. Butter the sliced rolls on both sides.
2. Whisk the eggs in an oven-safe dish.
3. Place the cheese, egg dish, and rolls into the air fryer. Make sure the buttered sides of the roll are facing upwards.
4. Adjust the air fryer to 390 degrees Fahrenheit. Cook for 6 minutes.
5. Place the egg and cheese between the pieces of roll. Serve warm.

Nutrition: Calories 212 Total Fat 11.2g Carbohydrates 9.3g Protein 12.4g

Peanut Butter and Banana Breakfast Sandwich

Preparation Time:4 Minutes

Cooking Time: 6 Minutes

Servings: 1

Ingredients:

- 2slices whole-wheat bread
- 1 tsp. sugar-free maple syrup
- 1 sliced banana
- 2tbsps. peanut butter

Directions:

1. Evenly coat each side of the sliced bread with peanut butter.
2. Add the sliced banana and drizzle with some sugar-free maple syrup.
3. Adjust the air fryer to 330 degrees Fahrenheit, then cook for 6 minutes. Serve warm.

Nutrition: Calories 211 Total Fat 8.2g Carbohydrates 6.3g Protein 11.2g

Morning Mini Cheeseburger Sliders

Preparation Time: 5 Minutes

Cooking Time: 10 Minutes

Servings: 6

Ingredients:

- 1 lb. ground beef
- 6slices of cheddar cheese
- 6dinner rolls
- Salt and Black pepper

Directions:

1. 1.Adjust the air fryer to 390 degrees Fahrenheit.
2. 2.Form 6 beef patties (each about 2.5 oz.) and season with salt and black pepper.
3. 3.Add the burger patties to the cooking basket and cook them for 10 minutes.
4. 4.Remove the burger patties from the air fryer; place the cheese on top of burgers, return to the air fryer and cook for another minute.
5. 5.Remove and put burgers on dinner rolls and serve warm.

Nutrition: Calories 262 Total Fat 9.4g Carbohydrates 8.2g Protein 16.2g

Breakfast Muffins

Preparation Time:3 Minutes

Cooking Time: 6 Minutes

Servings: 2

Ingredients:

- 2whole-wheat English muffins
- 4slices of bacon
- Pepper
- 2eggs

Directions:

1. Crack an egg each into ramekins, then season with pepper.
2. Place the ramekins in your preheated air fryer at 390 degrees Fahrenheit.
3. Allow cooking for 6-minutes with the bacon and muffins alongside.
4. Remove the muffins from the air fryer after a few minutes and split them.
5. When the bacon and eggs are done cooking, add two bacon pieces and one egg to each egg muffin. Serve when hot.

Nutrition: Calories 276 total Fat 12gCarbohydrates 10.2g Protein 17.3g

Tomato and Mozzarella Bruschetta

Preparation Time:5 Minutes

Cooking Time: 4 Minutes

Servings: 1

Ingredients:

- 6small loaf slices
- ½ cup tomatoes, finely chopped
- 3ounces (85 g) Mozzarella cheese, grated
- 1 tablespoon fresh basil, chopped
- 1 tablespoon olive oil

Directions:

1. Press Start/Cancel. Preheat the air fryer oven to 350 degrees Fahrenheit (177 degrees Celsius).
2. Put the loaf slices in the fry basket and insert the fry basket at mid position.
3. Select Air Fry, Convection, and set Time to 3 minutes.
4. Add the tomato, Mozzarella, basil, and olive oil on top.

5. Air fry for an additional minute before serving.

Nutrition: Calories 166 Fat 12g Carbohydrates 11g Protein 3g

All-in-One Toast

Preparation Time:10 Minutes

Cooking Time: 10 Minutes

Servings: 1

Ingredients:

- 1 strip bacon, diced
- 1 slice 1-inch-thick bread
- 1 egg
- Salt and freshly ground black pepper, to taste
- ¼ cup grated Colby cheese

Directions:

1. Press Start/Cancel. Preheat the air fryer oven to 400 degrees Fahrenheit (204 degrees Celsius).
2. Place the bacon in the fry basket. Insert the fry basket at mid position.
3. Select Air Fry, Convection, and set Time to 3 minutes, shaking the basket once or twice while it cooks. Remove the bacon to a paper towel-lined plate and set aside.
4. Use a sharp paring knife to score a large circle in the middle of the bread slice,

cutting halfway through but not through to the cutting board. Press down on the circle in the center of the bread slice to create an indentation.

5. Transfer the slice of bread, hole side up, to the fry basket. Crack the egg into the center of the bread and season with salt and pepper.

6. Adjust the air fryer oven temperature to 380 degrees Fahrenheit (193 degrees Celsius) and air fry for 5 minutes. Sprinkle the grated cheese around the bread's edges, leaving the yolk's center uncovered, and top with the cooked bacon. Press the cheese and bacon into the bread lightly to help anchor it to the bread and prevent it from blowing around in the air fryer oven.

7. Air fry for two more minutes, just to melt the cheese and finish cooking the egg. Serve immediately.

Nutrition: Calories 243 Fat 14.5g Carbohydrates 15.4g Protein 12.6g

Jalapeño Tacos with Guacamole

Preparation Time:10 Minutes

Cooking Time: 30 Minutes

Servings: 3

Ingredients:

- 3soft taco shells
- 1 cup kidney beans, drained
- 1 cup black beans, drained
- ½ cup tomato puree
- 1 fresh jalapeño pepper, chopped
- 1 cup fresh cilantro, chopped
- 1 cup corn kernels
- ½ tsp ground cumin
- ½ tsp cayenne pepper
- Salt and black pepper to taste
- 1 cup grated mozzarella cheese
- Guacamole to serve

Directions:

1. In a bowl, add beans, beans, tomato puree, chili, cilantro, corn, cumin, cayenne, salt and pepper; stir well. Spoon the mixture onto one half of the taco, sprinkle the

cheese over the top and fold over. Spray the frying basket, and lay the tacos inside. Cook for 14 minutes at 360 degrees Fahrenheit, until the cheese melts. Serve hot with guacamole.

Nutrition: Calories 419 Total Fat 14g Total Carbohydrates 39g Protein 33g

Mac and Cheese Balls

Preparation Time: 20 Minutes

Cooking Time: 25 Minutes

Servings: 6

Ingredients:

- ½ shredded pound mozzarella cheese
- 2 eggs
- 3 cup seasoned panko breadcrumbs
- Salt
- 2 tbsps. All-purpose flour
- 1 lb. Grated cheddar cheese
- 1 lb. Elbow macaroni
- 2 cup heated cream
- Pepper
- 2 tbsps. Unsalted butter
- 2 tbsps. Egg wash
- ½ lb. Shredded parmesan cheese

Directions:

1. Directions: are the macaroni in relation to the Directions: on the package.
2. Rinse with cold water and drain. Transfer to a bowl and set aside.

3. Melt butter in a saucepan over medium flame. Add flour and whisk for a couple of minutes. Stir the heated cream until there are no more lumps. Cook until thick. Remove from the stove. Stir in the cheeses until melted. Season with salt and pepper.

4. Top the cheese mixture onto the cooked macaroni. Gently fold until combined. Transfer to a shallow pan and refrigerate for 2 hours.

5. Use your hands to form meatball-sized balls from the mixture. Arrange them in a tray lined with wax paper. Freeze overnight.

6. Directions: are the egg wash by combining 2 tbsps. Of cream and eggs in a shallow bowl.

7. Dip the frozen mac and cheese balls in the egg wash and coat them with panko breadcrumbs. Gently press to make the coating stick.

8. Arrange them in the cooking basket. Cook for 8 minutes at 400 degrees.

Nutrition: Calories: 907 Fat: 423g Carbs: 874g

Protein: 499g

Cauliflower Fritters

Preparation Time:2 Minutes

Cooking Time: 13 Minutes

Servings: 4

Ingredients:

- Cauliflower Florets - 4 cups.
- Bread Crumbs - 1 cup
- Salt - 1 tsp.
- Butter - ¼ cup, melted.
- Buffalo sauce - ¼ cup

Directions:

1. Twitch by melting the butter in the microwave for 10 seconds.
2. Add the buffalo sauce into the butter and whisk well.
3. Hold each cauliflower by its stem and dip it into the mixture.
4. Next, coat the cauliflower into the bread crumbs.
5. Place the coated cauliflowers into the air fryer.
6. Cook 400 degrees F for 12 minutes.

7. After 7 minutes, toss the cauliflowers and cook for another 6 minutes.
8. Once done, serve hot and enjoy or with your favorite dip.

Nutrition: Calories: 80 Fats: 6g Protein: 6g Carbs: 1g

Loaded Tater Tot Bites

Preparation Time:5 Minutes

Cooking Time: 20 Minutes

Servings: 6

Ingredients:

- 24 tater tots, frozen
- 1 cup Swiss cheese, grated
- Six tablespoons Canadian bacon, cooked and chopped
- 1/4 cup Ranch dressing

Directions:

1. Spritz the silicone muffin cups with non-stick cooking spray. Now, press the tater tots down into each cup.
2. Divide the cheese, bacon, and Ranch dressing between tater tot cups.
3. Cook in the preheated Air Fryer using 395 degrees for 10 minutes. Serve in paper cake cups. Bon appétit!

Nutrition: Calories 164 Fat 7g Carbs 2g Protein 3g Sugar 8g

Italian-Style Tomato-Parmesan Crisps

Preparation Time: 5 Minutes

Cooking Time: 20 Minutes

Servings: 4

Ingredients:

- 4 Roma tomatoes, sliced
- Two tablespoons olive oil
- Sea salt and white pepper, to taste
- One teaspoon Italian seasoning mix
- Four tablespoons Parmesan cheese, grated

Directions:

1. Begin by preheating your Air Fryer, then set it to 350 degrees F. Generously grease the Air Fryer basket with nonstick cooking oil.

2. Toss the sliced tomatoes with the remaining ingredient. Transfer them to the cooking basket without overlapping.

3. Cook in the warmed Air Fryer for 5 minutes. Shake the cooking basket and cook an additional 5 minutes. Work in batches.

4. Serve with Mediterranean aioli for dipping, if desired. Bon appétit!

Nutrition: Calories 90 Fat 2g Carbs 7g Protein 8g Sugar 1g

Baked Cheese Crisps

Preparation Time:5 Minutes

Cooking Time: 15 Minutes

Servings: 4

Ingredients:

- 1/2 cup Parmesan cheese, shredded
- 1 cup Cheddar cheese, shredded
- One teaspoon Italian seasoning
- 1/2 cup marinara sauce

Directions:

1. Begin by preheating your Air Fryer and set it to 350 degrees F. Place a piece of parchment paper in the cooking basket.
2. Mix the cheese with the Italian seasoning.
3. Add around one tablespoon of the cheese mixture (per crisp to the basket, making sure they are not touching—Bake for 6 minutes or until browned to your liking.
4. Work in batches and place them on a large tray to cool slightly. Serve with the marinara sauce. Bon appétit!

Nutrition: Calories 198 Fat 17g Carbs 7g Protein 12g Sugar 4g

Puerto Rican Tostones

Preparation Time:5 Minutes

Cooking Time: 15 Minutes

Servings: 2

Ingredients:

- One ripe plantain, sliced
- One tablespoon sunflower oil
- A pinch of grated nutmeg
- A pinch of kosher salt

Directions:

- Toss the plantains with the oil, nutmeg, and salt in a bowl.
- Cook in the preheated Air Fryer at 400 degrees F for 10 minutes, shaking the cooking basket halfway through the cooking Time.
- Regulate the seasonings to taste and serve immediately.

Nutrition: Calories 151 Fat 1g Carbs 29g Protein 6g Sugar 17g